'/13

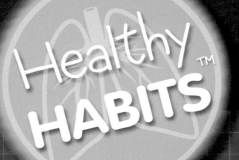

Sexual Health
Understanding Your Body's Changes

Serena Gander-Howser

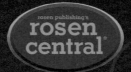

rosen publishing's
rosen
central

New York

Published in 2013 by The Rosen Publishing Group, Inc.
29 East 21st Street, New York, NY 10010

Copyright © 2013 by The Rosen Publishing Group, Inc.

First Edition

Library of Congress Cataloging-in-Publication Data

Gander-Howser, Serena.
Sexual health: understanding your body's changes/Serena Gander-Howser.—1st ed.
     p. cm.—(Healthy habits)
Includes bibliographical references and index.
ISBN 978-1-4488-6953-4 (library binding)
1. Sexual health. 2. Puberty. 3. Sex. 4. Health promotion. I. Title.
RA788.G28 2013
613.9—dc23

                                                                    2011052585

Manufactured in the United States of America

CPSIA Compliance Information: Batch #S12YA. For further information, contact Rosen Publishing, New York, New York, at 1-800-237-9932.

CONTENTS

Introduction

Sooner or later, it happens to every girl. You notice that you're growing taller and filling out. Your face breaks out, and you start growing hair where you never had it before. Your monthly menstrual cycle begins. You start paying attention to boys. Emotions seem more intense than they did before. All the girls at school are going through the same changes, too. Comparing yourself to them, you may wonder: Am I changing too quickly? Too slowly? What will I look like when I grow up? Will I be normal?

Sooner or later, it happens to every boy. You notice changes "down there," and your private parts seem to take on a mind of their own. You get taller, and your muscles get bigger. You start to grow facial hair. You start getting crushes. You may feel like you're on an emotional roller coaster. Everyone tells you that you're becoming a man, but you just wonder: What kind of man will I be? Will I live up to others' expectations? What will I look like? Will I be normal?

Whether you are a boy or a girl, your hormones are going wild. There are chemicals coursing through your body, sending it the message that it's time to change, time to transform from a child into an adult. You're going through puberty.

Nobody ever said that growing up was easy. Puberty can be a confusing, embarrassing, frustrating, scary, bewildering, and exhausting time. Of course, you can also see puberty as an exciting time of discovery, growth, and new experiences. You'll make new friends, discover new interests, and learn new things.

Maybe because puberty is such a chaotic time, in the midst of all this confusion and excitement, teenagers can fall prey to serious health conditions. For example, many teens develop an unhealthy body image, which can lead to an eating disorder. Others experiment

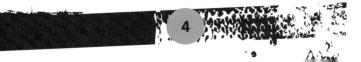

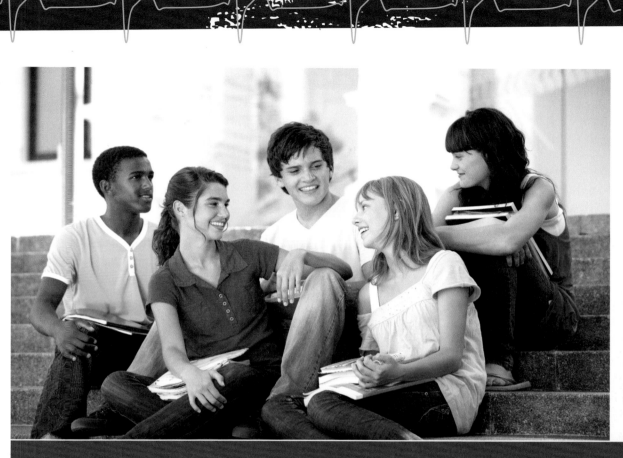

It's not always comfortable to talk about, but all teens go through puberty sooner or later.

with dangerous drugs, alcohol, or cigarettes. Teens who have unprotected sex may end up pregnant or with a sexually transmitted disease (STD). Still others get teased unnecessarily, simply because they can't or don't know how to keep acne or body odor under control. In some cases, teens who don't take care of themselves start on a road to lifelong health problems.

Luckily, there are simple things that you can do—eat right, exercise, stay clean, and stay calm—to help you survive puberty. This book will introduce habits that will help you stay healthy and develop confidence as you grow.

Chapter 1

Overview: Puberty

So what's the point of puberty, anyway? Why do people have to go through all these yucky, confusing changes in order to become grown-ups?

Biologically speaking, animals (including humans) reach adulthood when they are fully developed and able to reproduce. Many of the changes that you experience during puberty are getting you ready to have children one day. Others make you strong enough to care for your children or make you more easily recognizable as a man or a woman. As your body develops, you also become more emotionally and intellectually mature.

How Does Reproduction Work?

Why does your body need to change in order to have children? As you probably already know, having sex is nature's way of creating children. Of course, that is not its only purpose—grown-ups in committed relationships use sex to express their feelings of love and closeness for each other. But on a biological level, sexual intercourse is designed to deliver a man's sperm cells to a woman's egg cells. Once a sperm fertilizes an egg, it grows into a fetus and eventually into a baby.

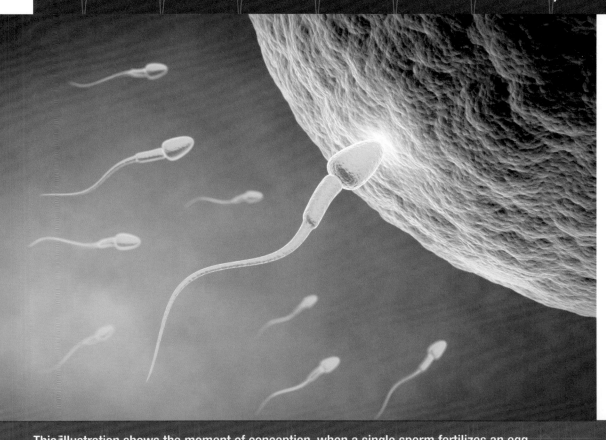

This illustration shows the moment of conception, when a single sperm fertilizes an egg.

n order for a man's sperm to reach a woman's egg, his penis must enter her vagina. In order to enter a vagina, a penis must become hard, which is called an erection. The vagina also changes, secreting lubricating fluid that makes it easier for the penis to enter. Once sufficiently stimulated, the erect penis will ejaculate, releasing a fluid called semen from its tip. Mature semen contains sperm, or male sex cells.

Roughly once a month, a woman ovulates, meaning that she releases an egg, or ovum, from one of her two ovaries (the organs that store a woman's eggs). The egg travels down the fallopian tube

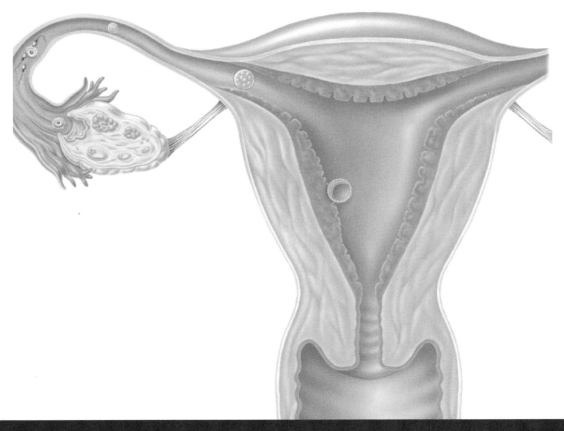

A woman's egg travels from the ovary (the yellow oval) down the fallopian tube. In this illustration, the egg is fertilized and then moves toward the uterus, which is cushioned with extra tissue.

and into her uterus, or womb. If a woman has unprotected sex (that is, sex without using birth control, such as the man wearing a condom), the man's sperm will swim to meet the egg, and a sperm may fertilize the egg.

A girl cannot get pregnant until she begins her menstrual cycle, which includes the monthly release of an egg, as well as other monthly changes that prepare her body for pregnancy. For example, the lining of the uterus thickens to prepare to receive a fertilized egg.

When Does Puberty Start?

Every person experiences puberty differently. It's normal for girls to start puberty as young as age ten, or not until they're fourteen or fifteen. Some girls experience early puberty around age eight. Girls typically develop faster than boys, who usually begin puberty between twelve and sixteen.

If you look around your class, chances are you will see that some students have already grown big and tall. Some girls have developed curves already, while some boys and girls haven't changed much at all. If you are worried that you are developing too early or too late, consult your doctor. Chances are, you are developing at a pace that is right for you.

If a woman releases an egg into her uterus but it is not fertilized, the body eventually expels the egg along with some of the blood-enriched lining of the uterus. This monthly flow of blood and tissues is commonly called a period. It is formally known as menstruation.

A boy cannot father a child until he is capable of getting an erection and creating and releasing sperm. In fact, during puberty, guys sometimes experience spontaneous erections that happen for no reason. They are just part of the body changing.

How Does Puberty Work?

Puberty begins when glands in the brain start releasing chemical signals through the bloodstream to the sex organs.

In boys' bodies, signals travel to the testes, the organs of the male body that produce sperm. The testes start producing a hormone

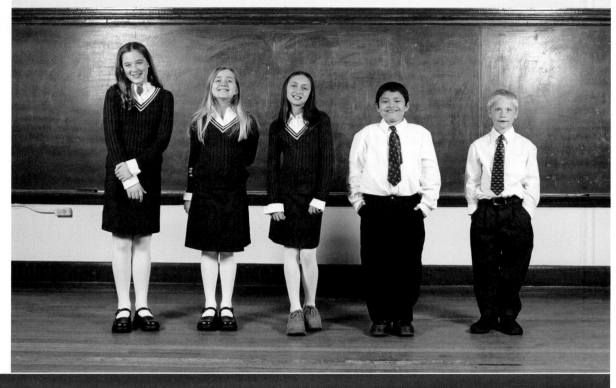

Every boy and every girl goes through puberty at his or her own pace. But in general, girls start to develop at an earlier age than boys.

called testosterone. Both men and women have testosterone in their bodies. But when a boy's body starts making testosterone during puberty, the hormone helps him build muscles and grow body and facial hair. It can also make a boy feel more aggressive, or more drawn to the people he is attracted to.

It's different for girls. At the beginning of puberty, a girl's ovaries start to produce the hormone estrogen. Both men and women have estrogen in their bodies. But the release of estrogen into a girl's system at the beginning of puberty influences her body in a special way. She starts growing breasts, developing curves, and menstruating.

Chapter 2

The Changes Girls Experience

Puberty doesn't happen to a girl overnight. First, the breasts start to develop. Next, a few hairs start to appear in the pubic region (above and around the genitals, or private parts). Eventually, a girl will get her period. Around that time or later, she will start to develop hips. When the long process of puberty is finally finished, she has the body of a mature woman.

Breasts

The first change that most girls experience is the development of firm, tender swellings underneath the nipples called breast buds. Most girls develop breast buds at about age ten or eleven, although it's perfectly normal for breasts to grow before or after this age.

Many girls worry that one of their breasts is growing faster than the other. This is normal. The breasts basically even out over time — although most women find that one of their breasts is slightly larger than the other. If your development continues to be very uneven for a long time, consult your doctor.

When girls become women and have children, they are able to breastfeed their babies if they choose to. As adults, women also need to start checking for breast cancer. According to the National Cancer

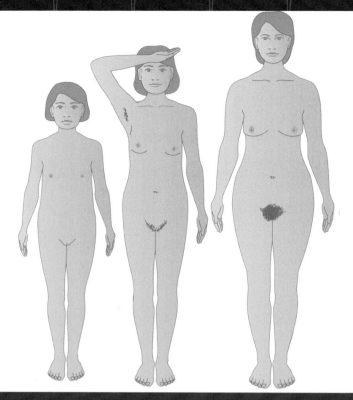

This illustration shows the stages of puberty that transform a girl's body into a woman's body. In the middle, you can see an adolescent female halfway through puberty.

Institute, breast cancer is the second most common form of cancer. Ask your doctor to show you how to perform a breast self-exam so that if you develop breast cancer, you can catch it early.

Bras

A hot topic among girls beginning puberty is bras. What's the right age to start wearing a bra? Do you have to wear one? The answers to these questions change from culture to culture, town to town, family to family, and girl to girl. Some girls never wear a bra; others wear a bra every day, only taking it off to go to bed. What you do is up to you.

If you engage in a lot of physical activities like sports or dance, you might want to wear a sports bra while working out. If you have large breasts, you may find it more comfortable to wear a structured bra for support.

The Right Size

Many girls waste a lot of time worrying about whether their breasts are too big or too small. Let's face it: our society is obsessed with women's bodies. Magazines show off celebrities' "beach bods," and makeover TV shows offer breast implants. To make matters more confusing, large breasts will be fashionable one

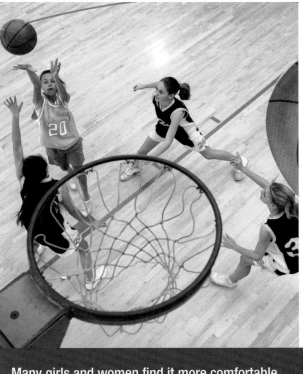

Many girls and women find it more comfortable to wear a sports bra when playing sports, jogging, dancing, mountain biking, or participating in other physical activities.

year, and small-breasted models will be all the rage the next.

Some girls are tempted to take supplements to make their breasts grow bigger. Be warned: these products are useless at best and dangerous at worst. Some women even undergo surgical breast augmentation or breast reduction. Doctors don't recommend getting cosmetic surgery before your body has finished growing (which may not be until your mid-twenties). Breast implants can create health problems later in life, especially if they rupture, or break open. Also, most women will need to have their implants replaced at some point, requiring another surgery.

It is easier and safer to love the body you have than try to change it through surgery, supplements, or extreme dieting.

Hair and Hips

Around the time that girls start developing breasts, pubic hair begins growing around the vulva (the female outer sex organs). The first of these hairs to appear are usually straight, thin, and fair. As a girl gets older, the hairs get thicker, darker, and curlier.

Girls will also start to notice hair growing underneath their armpits and on their arms and legs. If you, like many American women, decide to shave your armpits and legs, make sure that an older woman you trust shows you how to shave safely.

During puberty, girls' hips widen and become rounder. Some new weight appears on the thighs and rear end. As the hips widen, the waist narrows in proportion to the hips.

Getting Your Period

A period is part of the monthly menstrual cycle. About once a month, women ovulate; one of the two ovaries releases an egg, which travels down a fallopian tube and into the uterus. Once released, the egg may join with a sperm, become fertilized, and come to rest in the uterus. A fertilized egg must be nourished and cushioned. So every month, the body reinforces the walls of the uterus with blood and other nutrient-rich tissues.

However, the egg can only be fertilized within a certain window of time. If the egg is not fertilized, the body releases the egg along with the blood and tissue lining the uterus. This flow is called a period.

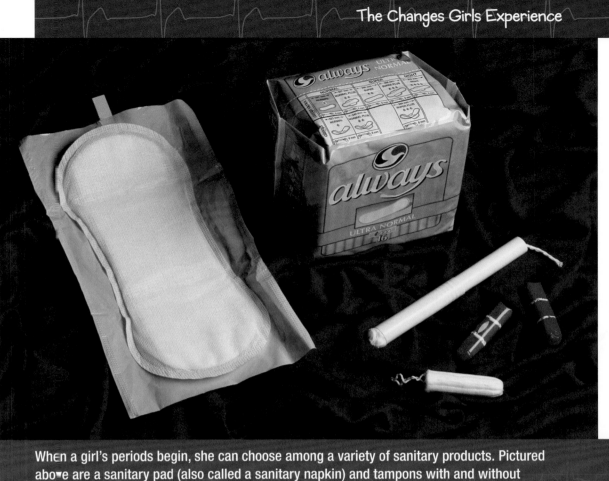

When a girl's periods begin, she can choose among a variety of sanitary products. Pictured above are a sanitary pad (also called a sanitary napkin) and tampons with and without applicators.

Most females' periods last for three to five days. However, every woman's period is different, and it can change over time. A girl might experience a light flow one month and a heavy flow the next. Periods are generally about a month apart—that's why some people call a period a "monthly." Many women experience irregular periods that come more or less frequently. This is especially true for girls in the first years of their period. Some women keep track of their cycles so that they can predict which days of the month they can expect their period.

There's more to the menstrual cycle than just a period. Throughout the month, the hormones in a girl's body fluctuate, causing subtle changes in her body. For instance, a girl's breasts might swell slightly, she might become bloated, or she might experience some cramping before and during her period. However, some girls barely notice any changes.

Many (but certainly not all) women experience premenstrual syndrome, or PMS. Right before a woman gets her period, she may experience mood swings, fatigue, cramping, trouble sleeping, headaches, and cravings for certain types of food.

When Will I Get My Period?

Every girl wonders when she'll get her first period. Unfortunately, there's no way to tell for sure. Most girls first start to menstruate around eleven or twelve, although some start as early as ten or as late as fourteen. If you haven't gotten your first period by age fifteen, consult a doctor.

Once your menstrual cycle has established itself and become regular, changes in your cycle can signal health problems. For instance, your period can be thrown off if you exercise too much or get very stressed out. If your regular period suddenly becomes irregular, consult a doctor.

Keeping Clean During Your Period

Having your period isn't like urinating. You can't "hold in" your period! That's why women use sanitary products to avoid staining their clothes. The most popular sanitary products are tampons and pads. Most women use a combination of both.

Sanitary pads are bandage-like pads that are applied like stickers to the inside of your underwear. They absorb blood before it stains

Healthy Habits to Ease Period Pain

Not all girls experience discomfort or unpleasant physical or emotional symptoms around their periods. But if you do, staying healthy will make your period easier. Get enough sleep, drink plenty of water, eat healthy meals, and get regular exercise.

If you find that you get bloated around your period, avoid eating salty foods and snacks in the days leading up to your period. If you get a lot of cramps, stay away from caffeine before your period. While there are many over-the-counter medicines that claim to alleviate these symptoms, it's best to consult a doctor or pharmacist before taking any. One of the best cures for cramps is all-natural: a hot-water bottle or heating pad pressed against your lower stomach or back can go a long way in relieving cramps. Tell a trusted adult if these methods don't provide relief.

underpants and clothes. There are many different types of pads. Some are designed for very light flows; others are for heavy flows or overnight use. You will figure out which type of pad is right for you. Just change your pad every few hours, before it "bleeds through." After you remove a pad, wrap it in toilet paper or the wrapper from the new pad and throw it away in the garbage. (Pads can't be flushed down a toilet.)

Tampons are inserted into the vagina (the canal that leads from the vulva to the uterus) to absorb menstrual discharge. Read the directions carefully before using a tampon for the first time. You should also ask a woman you trust to show you how to use it. Some tampons come with a plastic or cardboard applicator. The applicator is supposed to make it easier to insert the tampon. It should never be left inside you along with the tampon. Also, make sure to leave the tampon string hanging down once the tampon is inserted. The string will allow you to pull the tampon out.

Tampons are very convenient. Unlike pads, tampons allow you to go swimming during your period. However, it's important to pick the right tampon and change your tampon frequently. Change it as soon as it gets soaked through, or about every three to four hours. Never leave a tampon in overnight. Choose a tampon whose absorbency matches your flow—a light tampon for light days or a "super," high-absorbency tampon if your flow is extremely heavy. Along with the tampon, you can also use a panty liner (an extremely thin pad) as backup protection.

If you leave a tampon in for too long, or you routinely use tampons that are more absorbent than needed, you could develop a rare but serious condition called toxic shock syndrome (TSS). TSS causes rashes, vaginal discharge, dizziness and fainting, fever, and muscle pains. The link between tampon use and TSS is not clearly understood. However, research shows that the risk of tampon-related TSS is associated with absorbency: the higher the absorbency, the higher the risk; the lower the absorbency, the lower the risk. That's why you should always use the lowest absorbency tampon appropriate for your menstrual flow.

Chapter 3

The Changes Boys Experience

For boys, puberty usually begins with a growth spurt. A boy might grow from 2 to 2½ inches (approximately 5 to 6 centimeters) in a year. Next, he starts to notice changes in his genitals, or private parts. First the testicles and then the penis will grow. From there, the changes will keep on coming.

Changes in Sexual Organs

During puberty, a boy's genitals will grow and change. It might sound funny or gross, but facts are facts: the penis will grow bigger and longer. The testicles will grow larger. The skin of the scrotum—the sac of skin around the testicles—will become thinner and darker, and the testicles will hang lower.

A lot of preteen and teenage guys worry that their penis won't reach the "right" size. Remember, all guys develop on their own time-line. You may not finish developing until you are in your twenties. That's why it's important not to experiment with vitamins, supplements, pumps, or other silly "medical" solutions that claim to enhance penis size. Every guy has a different body. There's no such thing as a "right" size. However you end up developing will be right for you.

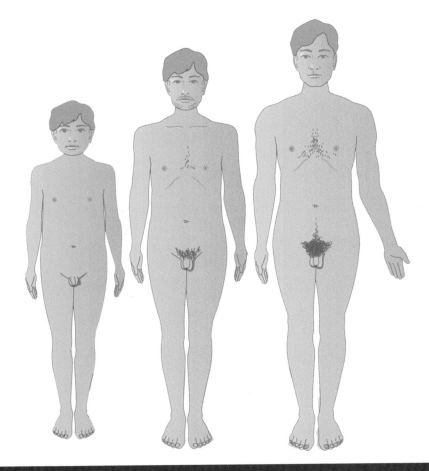

This graphic shows the changes that occur in a boy's body as he becomes a man. In the middle is a male teenager midway through puberty.

Taking Care of Your Private Parts

Part of staying healthy and happy as a teenager is learning to take care of your private parts. How you take care of yourself depends on whether or not you are circumcised. Circumcision is the removal of the foreskin, either for religious purposes or due to medical and hygienic concerns. There are millions of both circumcised and uncircumcised men in North America.

The penis should be washed regularly. If you are uncircumcised, it's important to wash underneath the foreskin as you grow older, sweat more, and start to produce and ejaculate sperm. Roll the foreskin back when you are bathing. Use soap and water to clean any secretions or "white stuff" off yourself. Remember to rinse. Many boys have tight foreskins, meaning the foreskin is so tight that they have difficulty rolling it back. If you have this problem, ask your doctor for advice. He or she may recommend gentle stretching exercises or prescribe a steroid cream that can help.

Athletic Supporters

As genitals grow bigger, lower, and more sensitive, it becomes important to protect them. When playing sports or exercising, males run the risk of twisting or otherwise damaging their genitals. Luckily, there are a number of ways to keep your sensitive parts secure and comfortable.

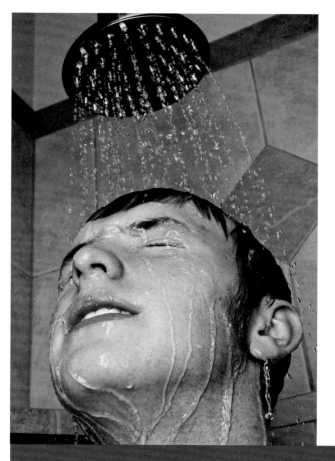

Showering every day and washing thoroughly is an important way to stay clean and healthy during puberty.

Today, jockstraps, or athletic supporters, are considered a bit old fashioned, but they are effective. An athletic supporter consists of a waistband (usually elastic) with a support pouch for the genitals, with straps attached to the legs to keep the pouch in place. You can also find supportive underwear, such as support briefs, jock briefs, and dance belts. Some athletic supporters come with padded or plastic protective cups. These come in handy if you're playing a particularly rough sport.

Erections

An erection is what happens when the spongy tissue of the penis fills with blood; the penis becomes stiff, sticking out from the body. Usually, an erection is caused by an arousing touch, situation, sight, or thought. But during puberty, when the body is full of hormones, boys will sometimes get erections for no reason at all. These are called spontaneous erections. They can be embarrassing and upsetting, but they are completely normal. If you experience one in public, relax and try to think about something else. Stand or sit in a way that hides the erection.

When a boy starts getting erections and ejaculating (releasing fluid called semen from the penis), the semen is clear. This is because the body hasn't created sperm yet. When the body starts producing sperm, the semen becomes white.

Some men and boys tend to get erections in the morning. Some stop experiencing this in their twenties; others never do. Either way is normal. Erection and ejaculation can also happen during sleep. When a boy experiences erection and ejaculation in his sleep, it's called a nocturnal emission, or "wet dream." Like spontaneous erections, wet dreams are a normal part of development during puberty.

Facial Hair

Later in puberty, males begin growing facial hair. They have the choice of growing out their facial hair or shaving it off. If you decide to shave, ask a parent or another grown-up you trust to show you the basics.

Electric razors are easier and safer to use. Plus, you don't need to use shaving cream with electric razors. If you use a regular razor, make sure you prepare your face with water or shaving cream. If you shave your face dry, you may cut yourself or irritate your skin. At first, shave in short strokes, going in the direction the hair grows in. When hairs first come in, shaving against the direction of hair growth could irritate your skin.

Many boys look forward to growing facial hair. Some experiment with growing a moustache or a beard.

Growing Muscles

During puberty, you will build bigger muscles, or "fill out." This will happen naturally. Working out can help a little—but don't go overboard! If you work out too hard before your body is ready, you might do more harm than good. If you want to lift weights, consult a coach who knows how to design a safe weight-lifting program for teens.

Breasts?

Some boys find that their breasts start to grow and swell slightly during puberty. This is a perfectly normal side effect of the hormones changing the body during puberty. If this happens to you, you'll probably worry that you are developing "man boobs." Don't worry—you're not. In a few weeks or months, the swelling will go away.

Body Hair

During adolescence, boys start growing hair in places where they never had it before. First, boys grow a few straight pubic hairs around the genitals. By the end of puberty, males will have dark, curly pubic hair covering the pubic region.

Boys also start to grow hair under their arms, and then on their legs and arms. Many grow hair on their chests and backs. Some guys prize a clean-shaven chest; others believe that a hairy chest is a sign of manliness. Your body and your hair are unique, so be proud.

Your Changing Voice

During puberty, a boy's voice will begin to "break," which means it will change from a high pitch to a low pitch and back again. This can be embarrassing, but there's nothing a boy can do about it. After a few months, his voice will settle into a lower register.

Why do boys' voices change? The sounds of the voice are created when air passes through the vocal cords, which are located in the larynx, or voice box, at the top of the trachea (windpipe). These cords make a lower sound when they are loose and relaxed and a higher sound when they are short and tight. During puberty, testosterone makes the larynx grow bigger, and the vocal cords grow longer and thicker, causing the voice to drop.

When the larynx grows bigger, it might start to jut out from the neck. This projection is known as an Adam's apple.

Chapter 4

Changes Everybody Experiences

All adolescents go through a growth spurt, get pimples, start producing body odor, and experience upheavals in their emotional lives. Both boys and girls need to know how to cope with these changes.

Growth Spurt

Boys and girls experience growth spurts. An adolescent might grow from 2 to 10 inches (5 to 25 cm) in a very short time. Girls generally go through a growth spurt between ages eight and thirteen, and most boys experience theirs between ten and fifteen. As teens shoot upward, they often become skinnier and lankier because they're growing so quickly that they don't have time to put on extra weight.

Because they're growing so quickly, many teens go through an "awkward phase." Their hands and feet seem too big for their bodies, and they become clumsier. Eventually, boys and girls reach their adult height and "grow into" their new bodies.

During your growth spurt, you will need to stretch before and after working out. Your bones might be growing faster than your tendons and ligaments, making these soft tissues tighter and more prone to injury.

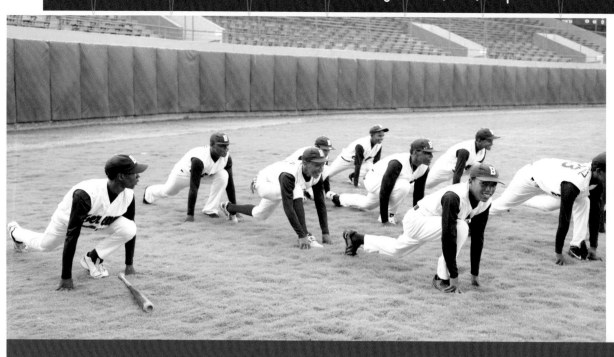

During your growth spurt, you might feel uncoordinated and clumsy. Remember to stretch before you work out or play sports.

Acne

One of the most unpleasant side effects of puberty is acne, a condition that makes blemishes like pimples, blackheads, whiteheads, and nodules appear on the face and other parts of the body.

Teens going through puberty get acne because their skin is changing. Pores and hair follicles contain sebaceous glands, which secrete oil called sebum. Sebum keeps hair shiny and skin moisturized. During puberty, hormones make the sebaceous glands work overtime. If the skin produces too much oil, the oil can clog pores, perhaps trapping dirt or dead skin inside and creating a pimple. Bacteria sometimes get trapped inside a clogged pore; the bacteria then reproduce and cause more acne.

Romantic Feelings

As you go through puberty, you will probably get a crush on, or have strong romantic feelings for, a special person. It's normal to feel confused, nervous, and unsure how to act around your crush. Remember to follow the golden rule: Don't be mean to crushes because you're scared of them, and don't hate them if they don't have the same feelings.

If the person you like *does* like you back, it can be very exciting. However, don't give up the rest of your life to date him or her. Suddenly dropping friends and activities and ignoring schoolwork in order to spend more time with a crush is a recipe for disaster.

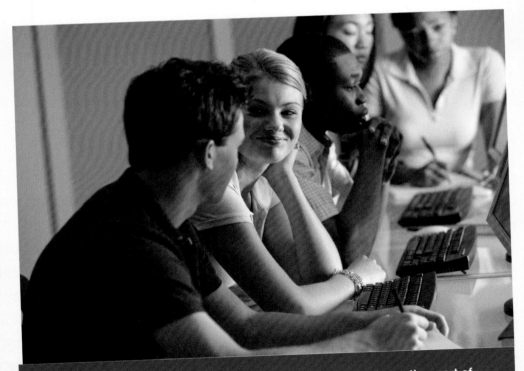

Starting to get crushes—experiencing romantic feelings—is another part of puberty. The hormones coursing through your body can make your attraction feel strong and even all-consuming.

Avoid acne by washing your face regularly with mild soap and warm water. Girls prone to breakouts should use oil-free makeup and skin products. Don't pick at or "pop" pimples. Pimples should go away on their own. If you pick at them or pop them, you could create tiny but lasting scars on your face.

There are many over-the-counter face washes and creams that can control acne. However, if you use them too much, you run the risk of drying out the skin and making matters worse. If your acne becomes severe, consult a dermatologist.

During puberty, your sebaceous glands will also make your hair shinier, maybe even greasier. It's important that you start to wash your hair more often than you did when you were younger. Avoid using products that add oil to your hair.

Body Odor

At some point during puberty, you'll start sweating more. You'll also notice a new smell under your armpits and around your private parts after you work out. This smell is called body odor, or "BO."

Why do we get BO? We're all born with two different types of sweat glands. Eccrine glands cool down the body with salty sweat. These glands are already active when you're a child. Apocrine glands release a substance that regulates your perspiration. The body has the most apocrine glands in the armpits and around the genitals. Children don't produce much apocrine sweat, but teens going through puberty produce a lot. The bacteria that naturally live on the skin love to feed off apocrine sweat. When they break down your sweat, they leave behind nasty-smelling chemicals.

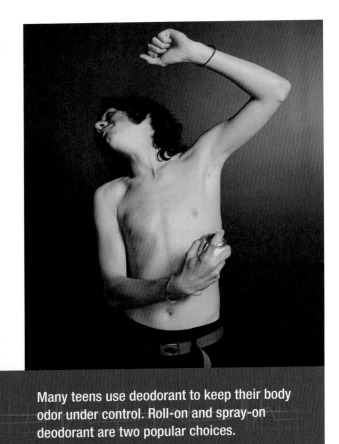

Many teens use deodorant to keep their body odor under control. Roll-on and spray-on deodorant are two popular choices.

You can fight BO by taking regular showers and washing with antibacterial soap. Always wear clean clothes: bacteria love dirty clothes and other moist environments.

Many people use deodorant, a product applied to the armpits to mask your scent with the scent of the deodorant. Others use an antiperspirant, which reduces sweating and helps keep bacteria under control. Many drugstore products are a combination of both.

Hormones and Emotions

The hormones coursing through your body change the way you think and feel during puberty. Your emotions may feel more intense. You might swing quickly from one powerful emotion to another, furious one minute and goofy the next.

Since everything in your life is changing so quickly, it's normal to feel a little sensitive. Many teenagers become very concerned with how their friends see them. Unfortunately, some teens play power games with each other, excluding or turning on each other for no reason. If you go through this, trust that it will pass. Find someone to talk to, like a friend, sibling, parent, or other adult you trust. Expressing your feelings can help you feel less alone.

30

If someone says or does something that makes you mad, count to ten before you respond. If you suddenly feel overwhelmed with sadness or frustration, give yourself a time-out. Listen to music. Take a walk. Express your negative emotions positively through art, writing, dance, or physical activity.

MYTHS and FACTS

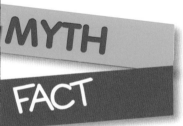

Periods are always very painful for girls.

Every woman's period is different. While some girls experience painful cramping and bloating during their periods, others barely notice their periods at all.

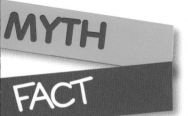

If you're a guy, you can buy products that will make your penis bigger.

The pills, lotions, pumps, extender devices, and exercises that claim to increase penis size are scams. At best, they don't work; at worst, they can harm your body.

MYTH

It's gross and abnormal to have feelings for people of the same sex.

FACT

It is both normal and natural to experience feelings for people of the same sex. During puberty, your hormones are going wild, and you

(Continued on next page)

(Continued from previous page)

will experience all sorts of new feelings. Feeling attracted to somebody of the same sex does not necessarily mean that you are gay, unless your feelings are very consistent and very strong over a long period of time. If this is the case for you, it's important for you to know that it's perfectly OK to be gay. While not everyone is accepting of homosexuality, there are millions of people all over the world who accept this sexual orientation as perfectly normal. It's important to find some-one supportive you can talk to so that you don't feel alone. People who can support you include a doctor or other health professional, a counselor or therapist, or an accepting relative or friend.

Chapter 5

What Can Go Wrong

Most teens make it through puberty basically unscathed, except for a few embarrassing experiences or a couple of stupid mistakes. But some kids contend with serious health issues during their teen years. Coping with your body's changes may include dealing with some serious health problems, especially if you're not careful.

Health Issues for Girls

Girls face special health challenges as they grow into young women. Some of these challenges are physical. Others are bad habits—like excessive dieting—that can develop into serious health problems if left unchecked.

Changes in the female body during puberty make girls more vulnerable to certain problems in and around the genitals. Here are a few to look out for.

Yeast Infections

A microscopically small fungus called *Candida albicans* often causes vaginal yeast infections. This microorganism lives on the surface of the skin, inside the mouth, in the digestive tract, and on other points on and inside the body. Sometimes, the yeast living on us and in us can multiply, get out of control, and cause

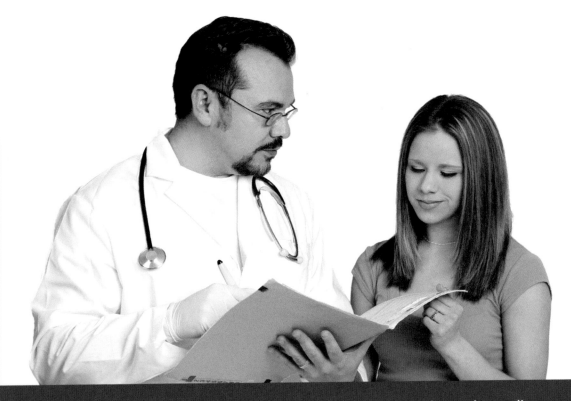

If you experience changes in your body that are painful or seem abnormal, consult your doctor.

infections. Yeast infections are of special concern for girls because this fungus thrives in warm, moist areas like the vagina.

Symptoms of a vaginal yeast infection include itching, burning, and swollen genitals; pain when urinating; and white or watery fluid discharging from the vagina. If you are experiencing your first infection, see a doctor for advice.

To prevent yeast infections, keep your private parts clean and dry and wear comfortable cotton underwear. Also avoid using scented feminine products since they can upset the natural balance of micro-organisms in the vagina.

Urinary Tract Infections (UTIs)

Urinary tract infections are also common. Any part of the urinary tract, including the kidney, the ureters (the tubes that take urine from the kidneys to the bladder), the bladder, or the urethra (the tube that empties the bladder) can be infected. Both males and females can get urinary tract infections, but UTIs are far more common in females. Women have a shorter urethra that gets infected more easily.

Symptoms of a UTI include foul-smelling, cloudy, or bloody urine. Urination is often painful, and it may be harder for you to "hold in" your urine. A UTI is sometimes accompanied by a low fever and cramps in the lower back.

Polycystic Ovary Syndrome (PCOS)

PCOS stands for polycystic ovary syndrome. This disorder involves an imbalance in a woman's hormones. In women with PCOS, the ovaries make more androgens than normal. Androgens are male hormones that females also create, but high levels of them affect a woman's ovulation.

PCOS-related problems include cysts (small sacs of fluid) on the ovaries. The syndrome can also change a woman's menstrual cycle, cause skin problems such as acne, cause unwanted hair growth, and lead to fertility problems (difficulties becoming pregnant). PCOS is more common than you might think: according to Children's Hospital Boston, nearly one out of every ten young women has PCOS.

PCOS usually appears after a girl starts her menstrual cycle. The most common symptoms include irregular periods, patches of dark skin, extra hair growing on the face or body, and weight gain. Only a doctor can diagnose PCOS, so if any of these symptoms apply to you, visit a health care provider.

Endometriosis

Severe menstrual cramps or mysterious pains in the pelvis can be signs of endometriosis. Sometimes, the tissue that normally lines the uterus is found in other parts of the body, such as the ovaries, fallopian tubes, or parts of the bladder or rectum. This tissue causes mysterious pains, cramping, and sometimes abnormal bleeding. See your doctor to diagnose endometriosis, get treatment, and learn how to keep the pain under control.

Eating Disorders

There's nothing wrong with healthy dieting or exercise to lose a little weight. However, when a girl becomes convinced that she's "too fat" no matter how much weight she loses, and when her obsession with thinness starts affecting her health, she's no longer just watching her weight—she's sick. She has developed an eating disorder. Eating disorders can lead to major medical problems and even death.

There are several kinds of eating disorders. People with anorexia nervosa obsessively starve themselves to lose weight. Although anorexia affects men as well as women, 85 to 95 percent of people with anorexia are women, according to the U.S. Department of Health and Human Services. Anorexics see themselves as fat, no matter how thin they are. They simply can't see how emaciated and sickly they have become. If the problem goes far enough, an anorexic will stop getting her period and become very constipated. Her skin will dry out and become yellow, and her hair and nails will grow brittle. In very severe cases, she may permanently damage her brain, heart, and other organs. She may even die.

Another common eating disorder is bulimia nervosa. People afflicted with this disease are called bulimics. Bulimics binge by eating large amounts of food. Then they get rid of the extra calories by vomiting or taking laxatives (known as purging) or doing extreme amounts of exercise. Bulimia has serious health consequences. Symptoms may include sore throat, rotting and decaying teeth (weakened by exposure to stomach acid), stomach problems, dehydration, and heart problems.

When a person overeats obsessively without purging, this is called binge eating disorder. People with binge eating disorder will often become overweight or obese, creating health problems like high blood pressure and heart disease.

If your relationship with food is getting out of control, seek help right away. This is

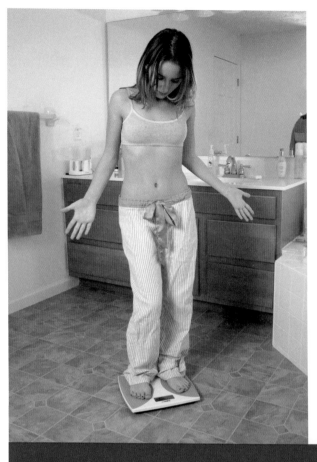

Teen girls, who are often insecure about their changing bodies, are especially vulnerable to eating disorders.

especially true if there is a history of eating disorders in your family. Living with an eating disorder for too long could literally cost you your life.

Overexercise: The Female Athlete Triad

Regular exercise is an important part of a healthy lifestyle. But some girls who play a lot of sports or exercise very intensely are at risk of developing a problem known as the female athlete triad. The female athlete triad consists of three different conditions, which can be experienced separately or all together:

- **Disordered eating.** With this condition, a girl purposely tries to lose weight in order to succeed in a specific sport, such as track, ballet, or gymnastics.
- **Amenorrhea.** This occurs when a girl is exercising so intensely and eating so little that her estrogen drops and her periods become irregular or stop.
- **Osteoporosis.** With this condition, a girl's bones don't develop the strength and density that they should, and they become weak and brittle.

To avoid the female exercise triad, eat regular meals, get plenty of calcium, don't overtrain, and keep track of your periods. If you train intensely and experience fatigue, stress fractures, muscle injuries, and/or irregular periods, visit your doctor.

Health Issues for Boys

Boys going through puberty face plenty of health challenges of their own. Unfortunately, male genitals are vulnerable to all sorts of infections, strains, and tears.

Urinary Tract Infections (UTIs)

Although many people think of urinary tract infections as a female problem, they also affect males. A UTI can develop in any part of the urinary system, including the urethra (the tube that empties urine from the bladder through the penis to the outside world), the bladder, and the kidneys. If you find that you need to urinate often, and if your urine burns, has a bad smell, or looks abnormal, see your doctor and ask if you might have a urinary tract infection.

Jock Itch

Jock itch is a red, scaly rash that breaks out around guys' groins. Sometimes, this rash is caused by irritated skin that has literally

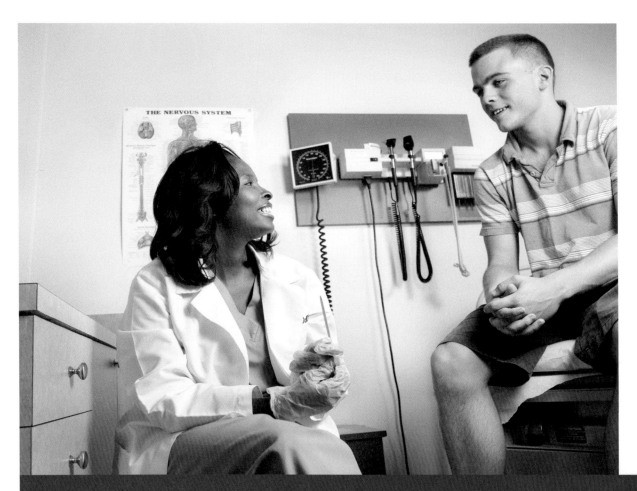

If you've noticed something is wrong around your genitals, don't let embarrassment stop you from seeking medical attention.

been rubbed the wrong way. Microorganisms called fungi that live in warm, moist places can infect the irritated skin. Jock itch can be contagious.

To avoid jock itch, keep yourself, your underwear, and your pants clean, dry, and fresh at all times. Take regular showers, and wear loose cotton underpants.

Testicular Torsion

The testes—the organs in a male's body that make sperm—hang somewhat loose inside the scrotum. They're connected to the body and to the scrotal wall by tissues, including the spermatic cord. But not all boys have the tissue that connects the testes to the scrotal wall. This means the spermatic cord may become twisted inside the scrotum, cutting off blood flow to the testicle. This can damage the testicle, and in some cases, surgery is needed to fix the problem. If left for too long, the testicle may need to be removed.

Guys from ten to twenty-five are at the greatest risk of experiencing testicular torsion. Torsion isn't always dramatic: very slight movements, gentle exercises, or even sleeping in a strange position can cause unexpected torsion. If you ever experience unexpected pain in the scrotum or testicles, get to a doctor right away. The chances of being able to fix the problem drop every hour that you delay getting help.

Body Image: Steroids and Eating Disorders

Not many people talk about it, but boys face body image problems just like girls do. Teen girls often feel pressure to look like the skinny models they see on TV, in magazines, and in movies. Similarly, the media typically show men who are tough, muscular, big, athletic, and strong. It's natural that boys want to live up to that image. So they are

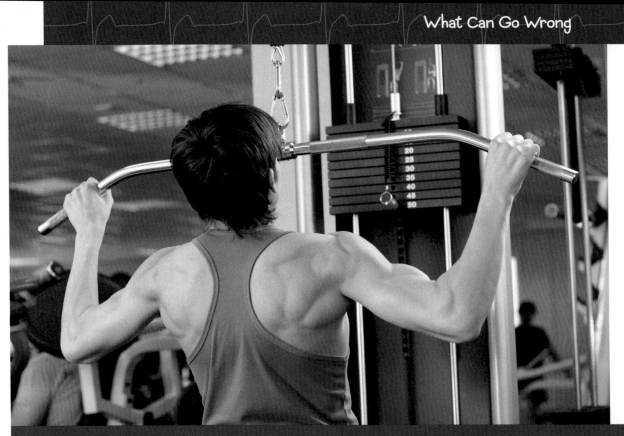

Weight training can be a great way for teen boys to strengthen muscles, gain confidence, and stay healthy. However, growing boys should avoid extreme bodybuilding or the use of risky supplements.

also vulnerable to eating disorders, including anorexia and bulimia. Binge eating disorder is especially common among teen boys.

Some young men become so obsessed with developing muscles that they start taking illegal anabolic steroids, synthetic hormones that help the body create bigger muscles. Professional athletes and bodybuilders are notorious for taking illegal steroids. These drugs have dangerous side effects, including stunted growth, hair loss, impotence (inability to get an erection), shrinking testicles, and difficulty urinating, along with other serious health problems. Also, injecting steroids and sharing needles puts people at risk of developing HIV or hepatitis B or C.

Sex and STDs

We can list sex among the risky behaviors that some teens engage in. You may already know that if you have sex—unprotected or protected—you run the risk of creating an unwanted pregnancy. But sex also puts you at risk of contracting a sexually transmitted disease (STD). You might have heard about HIV, the virus that causes AIDS. But there are many other very common STDs out there, including herpes, human papilloma virus (HPV), gonorrhea, chlamydia, syphilis, hepatitis, crabs, trichomoniasis, scabies, and chancroid.

You don't need to have vaginal intercourse (penis-in-vagina sex) to contract an STD. STDs can also be spread through other forms of sex, or even by having skin-to-skin contact with an infected area. Using protection such as condoms can help protect you from STDs. Remember: birth control pills will not protect you against STDs.

If you think you might have an STD, visit your doctor. You can ask your doctor to keep your visit confidential. If you think you might have an STD, do not have any sexual contact with anybody until a doctor has tested you.

Issues That Affect Both Boys and Girls

As you have seen, the teen years can be a treacherous time for boys and girls. Here are a few health problems that teenagers of both genders need to look out for.

Obesity

One health threat that increasingly affects Americans is obesity. For most people, obesity is preventable. When you eat extra calories that the body does not burn off through exercise, these calories are stored as fat. If you put on enough fat over time, you will become overweight or obese. According to a 2008 survey by the Centers for Disease

Control and Prevention (CDC), more than one-third of all American children and teens are overweight or obese.

Being overweight can be disastrous for your health. The more you weigh, the harder your body has to work to keep you going. The bones have to carry extra weight, and the heart has to work harder to pump blood. Other organs also have to work overtime. As a result, obesity can lead to fatigue, heart disease, arthritis, and hip problems. Obese youth can develop medical conditions that were once considered adult problems, including high cholesterol, type 2 diabetes, and high blood pressure.

Eating a healthy and balanced diet, avoiding guzzling sugary beverages and gorging on junk food, and getting plenty of exercise can prevent you from becoming obese. However, some people are born with a genetic predisposition to put on fat more quickly than others. If this applies to you, you will have to work harder than others to maintain a healthy weight.

Stress

Adolescence can be a stressful time. Teens stress out about their grades, relationships with friends and family, and futures. Living in a household that's struggling economically can cause a lot of stress, too.

Stress can damage your health. It can disrupt your sleep patterns and cause anxiety and depression. Stress may trigger panic attacks or episodes of irrational anger. Stress can also inspire people to "self-medicate" by using drugs or alcohol to unwind.

Fortunately, it's possible to develop healthy habits that will help you manage your stress. Make time to de-stress by expressing yourself in a journal, talking with friends, or taking some time off. You can also release tension by learning to meditate and stay healthy through exercise, balanced meals, and plenty of sleep.

Ten Great Questions
To Ask Your Health Care Provider

1 Am I developing too quickly or too slowly?

2 Am I overweight?

3 I've been experiencing some development recently that doesn't seem normal. If I tell you about it, would you promise to keep it confidential?

4 How can I make sure I get all the nutrients my body and brain need to grow?

5 My athletic performance is important to me, but so is my health. How can I make sure that I'm not overtraining?

6 What are some eco-friendly alternatives to tampons and pads?

7 I experience a lot of physical and emotional discomfort around my period. What are some ways to alleviate these symptoms?

8 I have irregular periods. Is that normal, or is it a sign of a health problem?

9 I'm interested in getting stronger. How can I build muscles in a safe way that won't damage my development?

10 How can I protect my private parts against damage while playing sports?

Chapter 6

How Healthy Habits Can Help You

There's so much about puberty that you can't control. But you can develop habits that will help you grow up healthier, happier, and ready to take on whatever challenges life throws your way.

Eat Healthy Foods

It's no secret that teenagers love fast food. Burgers, pizza, fries, chips, sodas, candy—teens know these foods are bad for them, but they crave them anyway. Companies design these foods so that you'll want to eat them again and again. The problem is, most of these foods are full of

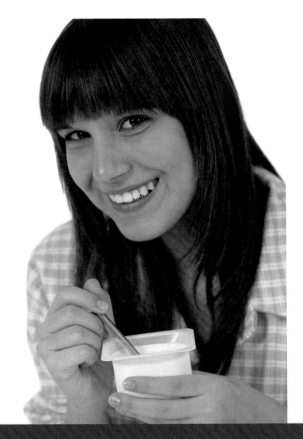

It's important for teenagers to eat a balanced and nutritious diet. Healthy snacks, like yogurt, help you stay strong and energetic.

empty calories. They cause you to put on weight but don't deliver any of the vitamins, minerals, and other nutrients that your body needs to grow strong.

If you live on fast food alone, you could become obese. If you don't get the vitamins and minerals you need, your brain will have a harder time making connections, meaning you'll have more difficulty thinking. So eating a balanced and nutritious diet is important!

Eating regular meals is crucial. Skipping meals can slow down your metabolism and make it harder for you to maintain a healthy weight. If you must skip a meal, replace it with a nutritious snack, not fast food. Grab a granola bar or a piece of fruit instead of chips. If you have a favorite fast-food spot, order the healthiest options on the menu.

Exercise

Exercise is one of the most important healthy habits. It burns extra calories to keep you at a healthy weight, it strengthens your bones, and it helps you fight disease. Exercise can also improve your mood. When you exercise vigorously, your body releases endorphins, chemicals that give you a sense of happiness and peace.

Doctors say that adolescents should engage in at least one hour of unbroken physical activity five times a week. You can dance, jog, play a sport—anything that increases your heart rate and breathing. Try switching off among different types of exercise. Aerobic exercise (running, biking, climbing stairs) should alternate with strength training (including sit-ups and pull-ups) and flexibility training (stretching).

Don't Smoke

Smoking tobacco is highly addictive and can seriously damage your lungs. In the short term, it will give you "smoker's cough," yellow your teeth, make your breath smell bad, and damage your body's ability to fight off sickness. In the long term, smoking may break down the tissues of your lungs, leading to emphysema and lung cancer.

The CDC reports that the negative consequences of smoking are responsible for one out of five deaths in the United States each year. If you've already started smoking, quit now. If you're not a smoker, don't start!

Don't Drink

It's legal for adults to drink alcohol, which leads many teens to believe that drinking is not really dangerous. When teens try drinking, they often engage in binge drinking, which can lead to injuries, alcohol poisoning, car crashes, and risky decisions. The CDC tells us that underage drinking is a major health problem in the United States. According to the agency, in 2008 underage drinking directly or indirectly led to over 190,000 trips to the emergency room in the United States.

According to the CDC, teens who drink are more likely to get bad grades, get arrested, abuse other drugs, and become involved in physical or sexual assaults. Plus, teens who start drinking before age fifteen are five times more likely to become alcoholics. Alcoholics and other heavy drinkers are at risk for developing cancer, cardiovascular problems, liver disease, impotence, neurological (brain-related) problems, and a host of other problems.

Don't Do Drugs

Most teens know that illegal drug use can lead to addiction and overdose. But they may be pressured to try drugs by friends who insist that drug use is "no big deal." The truth is, if you use illegal drugs during puberty, when your brain is still growing and developing, you could interfere with your brain's growth and even cause lasting brain damage.

Inform yourself about the risks of drug use. For instance, it's well known that excessive marijuana use leads to short-term memory loss. Crystal meth, if used enough, can cause symptoms that mirror Parkinson's disease. Even pills like pain relievers, tranquilizers, and attention deficit/hyperactivity disorder (ADHD) drugs can have very scary side effects if used without a doctor's prescription.

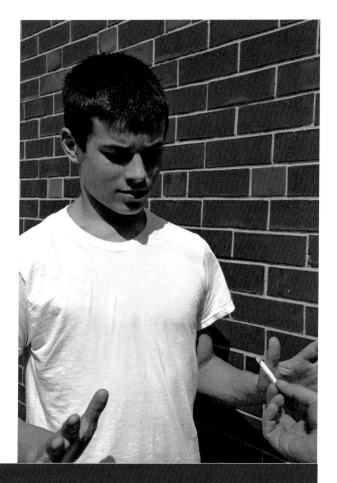

Contrary to what some teens believe, smoking marijuana is far from harmless. It can negatively affect the brain, heart, and lungs. Saying no to it is smart.

Be Smart About Sex

During puberty, hormones run wild. Some days it seems like all you can think about is getting close to that cute person you've got your eye on. But please don't rush into anything. STDs, unwanted pregnancies, heartbreak—the risks of teenage sex are real. Think hard before you decide to become sexually active.

Unprotected sex can lead to unwanted pregnancy. If you're a girl who is absolutely determined to become sexually active, look into birth control. Either the pill or another hormonal form of birth control, when used together with a condom, will protect you against unwanted pregnancy in most cases. However, it's important to remember that the only 100 percent effective form of birth control is abstinence.

Get Enough Sleep

When you're a teenager, your body is growing quickly. Most teens need a minimum of eight and a half hours of sleep a night. Getting enough sleep can be tough for teens because your changing body gravitates toward certain sleep habits. As you grow, you'll start wanting to stay up later and sleep later. This isn't laziness; it's a natural part of puberty. According to the Sleep Foundation, most teens have difficulty falling asleep before 11 PM.

Sleep deprivation can make you oversleep or fall asleep in class. It can also put you in a bad mood and make you clumsier. When you don't get enough sleep, it becomes harder to pay attention in class and remember what you've learned.

If, like many teens, you start school early in the day, you may need to find creative ways to get enough rest. Taking a nap after school can help. So can turning off all your electronics an hour before bedtime, avoiding caffeine or sugary beverages at night, and sleeping in a cool and dark room.

Unprotected sex also puts you at risk for contracting sexually transmitted diseases, which can be unpleasant at best (herpes, genital warts) and life-threatening at worst (HIV). Make it a rule to always use a condom. Although condoms do sometimes break or fail, using a condom is much, much safer than unprotected sex.

Accept Yourself as You Are

You may wonder if you'll ever live up to the standard set by models in glossy magazines. Models and movie stars are already blessed with conventionally good-looking faces and bodies. But the reality is, looking picture-perfect is still a full-time job for them. Many models and movie stars have personal trainers, intricately planned diets, personal hair and makeup artists, and even stylists to pick out all their clothes. Some go through expensive and dangerous plastic surgery or develop life-threatening eating disorders. Even after all that, they often have their photographs professionally altered and retouched.

It's important for you to know that there are many definitions of attractiveness around the world. In some cultures, a big belly on a man or woman is sexy. In some parts of Africa, women with a pear shape—big thighs and bottoms—are the ideal. Even in North America today, most men and women are attracted to people whose looks don't fit Hollywood's strict mold.

Seeing beauty in the body you were born with is much braver, stronger, and more satisfying than trying desperately to look like the cookie-cutter people you see on TV. You're the only person in the world who looks like you. Keep your own body healthy and strong. Celebrate it. Love it. Protect it. Don't starve it, exhaust it, or abuse it. Don't trash it with junk food, cigarettes, drugs, or alcohol. Stay healthy. Stay balanced. And follow your dreams.

absorbency A measure of how much liquid a substance can absorb.

acne An inflammatory disease of the skin in which the sebaceous glands become clogged and infected, often causing the formation of pimples, especially on the face, back, and chest.

alcohol poisoning A dangerous medical emergency that occurs when a person drinks too much, raising the level of alcohol in the bloodstream.

bacteria Microscopically tiny one-celled organisms that can reproduce quickly and thrive in all sorts of environments. Bacteria are responsible for a number of health conditions during adolescence, including acne and body odor.

binge To overindulge in an activity, especially eating or drinking.

birth control The prevention of pregnancy during sexual activity through the use of devices (such as condoms), drugs (such as birth control pills), or other techniques; contraception.

bloated Abnormally swollen with gas or fluid.

breast augmentation Surgery that artificially enlarges the breasts by inserting implants of saline or silicone inside them.

condom A protective covering for the penis that helps prevent disease, infection, and pregnancy.

cyst An abnormal sac of fluid or a fluid-filled cavity.

discharge A substance or material that is released from the body.

ejaculate To eject semen from the penis.

estrogen A hormone that mainly regulates the growth, development, and function of the female reproductive system, although it is also found in men.

fallopian tube One of two tubes that connect the ovaries to the uterus. Eggs must travel from the ovaries down the fallopian tube to the uterus.

fatigue Excessive sleepiness or tiredness.

foreskin The retractable sheath of skin that covers the tip of the penis in an uncircumcised male.

genitals A person's external reproductive organs.

hormone A chemical substance produced in the body that controls and regulates the activities of different parts of the body. Hormones affect many processes, including growth and development, sexual function, reproduction, mood, and metabolism.

larynx The voice box.

obese The medical term for being very overweight. Obesity is a medical problem because a person's excess fat can cause high blood pressure, diabetes, degeneration of bones and joints, and increased risk of cancer and stroke.

osteoporosis A disease that makes bones weak, brittle, and vulnerable to fractures. Teen girls can keep themselves from developing osteoporosis later in life by eating calcium-rich foods and exercising to increase bone strength.

ovary One of two reproductive organs in women that produce and release eggs (ova) and sex hormones.

ovulation The release of a mature egg (ovum) from an ovary.

Parkinson's disease A disease that causes the degeneration of the central nervous system, resulting in symptoms such as tremors and shaking, stiff muscles, inability to stay balanced, and slowness in movement.

premenstrual syndrome (PMS) The collective name for a number of physical and emotional symptoms experienced by some women prior to menstruation. Physical symptoms of PMS may include cramps or bloating. Emotional symptoms may include moodiness, depression, or irritability. Symptoms must be severe enough to interfere with a woman's life to be diagnosed as a medical condition.

scrotum The sac-like structure that holds the testicles, or testes.

semen The liquid released when the erect penis ejaculates. A mature man's semen contains millions of sperm, which are capable of fertilizing a woman's eggs.

testicle One of two reproductive male organs that produce sperm and testosterone. The testicles (also known as the testes) hang outside the male body, inside the scrotum.

testicular torsion A dangerous medical condition that develops when the spermatic cord twists, cutting off blood flow to the testicle.

testosterone The most important male sex hormone. Testosterone is found in men and women, but in men it helps regulate the growth and development of the reproductive organs, among other functions.

uterus The organ in the female body where children are conceived, gestate, and grow before birth; womb.

American Academy of Pediatrics (AAP)
141 Northwest Point Boulevard
Elk Grove Village, IL 60007-1098
(847) 434-4000
Web site: http://www.aap.org
The AAP is a professional association dedicated to the health, safety, and well-being of infants, children, and young adults. Its Web site provides information on pediatric issues and gives the public access to its publications.

American Medical Association (AMA)
515 North State Street
Chicago, IL 60654
(800) 621-8335
Web site: http://www.ama-assn.org
The AMA is a professional organization for physicians in the United States. It distributes information on issues important to physicians, patients, and the nation's health.

Boys & Girls Clubs of America
1275 Peachtree Street NE
Atlanta, GA 30309-3506
(404) 487-5700
Web site: http://www.bgca.org
Boys & Girls Clubs of America runs recreational clubs where children can learn, have fun, and feel a sense of belonging. Its programs include health and life skills initiatives that develop

young people's capacity to engage in healthy behaviors, set personal goals, and live successfully as self-sufficient adults.

Canadian Medical Association (CMA)
1867 Alta Vista Drive
Ottawa, ON K1G 5W8
Canada
Web site: http://www.cma.ca
(888) 855-2555
The CMA is a national association of physicians that advocates on behalf of its members and the public for access to high-quality health care. It also provides leadership and guidance to physicians.

Centers for Disease Control and Prevention (CDC)
1600 Clifton Road
Atlanta, GA 30333
(800) CDC-INFO [232-4636]
Web site: http://www.cdc.gov
The CDC collaborates to create the expertise, information, and tools that people and communities need to protect their health through health promotion; prevention of disease, injury, and disability; and preparedness for new health threats.

Children's Hospital Boston
300 Longwood Avenue
Boston, MA 02115

(800) 355-7944

Web site: http://www.childrenshospital.org

This pediatric hospital hosts a world-class research community. Its Division of Adolescent & Young Adult Medicine provides extensive health information for teens at http://www.youngwomenshealth.org and http://www.youngmenshealthsite.org.

Healthy Teen Network

1501 St. Paul Street, Suite 124

Baltimore, MD 21202

(410) 685-0410

Web site: http://www.healthyteennetwork.org

This national organization focuses on adolescent health and well-being with an emphasis on pregnancy prevention, teen pregnancy, and teen parenting. It builds capacity among professionals to help young people lead healthy sexual, reproductive, and family lives.

Planned Parenthood Federation of America

434 W. 33rd Street

New York, NY 10001

(212) 541-7800

Web site: http://www.plannedparenthood.org

This organization delivers reproductive health care, sex education, and information about reproductive health and family planning to millions of women, men, and young people worldwide. Its Web site contains comprehensive, medically accurate information for teens on puberty, their changing bodies, and sexuality.

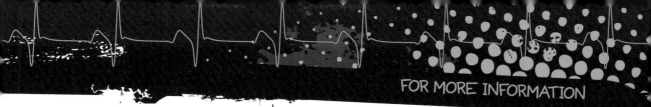

Society for Adolescent Health and Medicine (SAHM)
111 Deer Lake Road, Suite 100
Deerfield, IL 60015
(847) 753-5226
Web site: http://www.adolescenthealth.org
The SAHM is an international organization dedicated to advancing the health and well-being of adolescents through advocacy, clinical care, health promotion, professional development, and research.

Web Sites

Due to the changing nature of Internet links, Rosen Publishing has developed an online list of Web sites related to the subject of this book. This site is updated regularly. Please use this link to access the list:

http://www.rosenlinks.com/hab/sheal

Ashton, Jennifer, with Christine Larson. *The Body Scoop for Girls: A Straight-Talk Guide to a Healthy, Beautiful You*. New York, NY: Avery, 2009.

Attwood, Sarah. *Making Sense of Sex: A Forthright Guide to Puberty, Sex, and Relationships for People with Asperger's Syndrome*. Philadelphia, PA: Jessica Kingsley Publishers, 2008.

Belge, Kathy, and Marke Bieschke. *Queer: The Ultimate LGBT Guide for Teens*. San Francisco, CA: Zest Books, 2011.

Byers, Ann. *Frequently Asked Questions About Puberty* (FAQ: Teen Life). New York, NY: Rosen Publishing, 2007.

De la Bédoyère, Camilla. *Personal Hygiene and Sexual Health* (Healthy Lifestyles). Mankato, MN: Amicus, 2011.

Dunham, Kelli S. *The Boy's Body Book* (Boysworld). Kennebunkport, ME: Cider Mill Press, 2007.

Gray, Leon. *Puberty* (Being Healthy, Feeling Great). New York, NY: PowerKids Press, 2010.

Harris, Robie H., and Michael Emberley. *It's Perfectly Normal: A Book About Changing Bodies, Growing Up, Sex, and Sexual Health*. 3rd ed. Somerville, MA: Candlewick Press, 2009.

Holmes, Melisa, and Trish Hutchison. *Girlology's There's Something New About You: A Girl's Guide to Growing Up*. Deerfield Beach, FL: Health Communications, 2010.

Kershner, Tad. *Body Double: Understanding Physical Changes* (A Guy's Guide). Edina, MN: ABDO Publishing, 2011.

Levete, Sarah. *Coming of Age* (Journey of Life). New York, NY: Rosen Central, 2009.

Madaras, Lynda, and Area Madaras. *My Body, My Self for Boys*. Rev. 2nd ed. New York, NY: Newmarket Press, 2007.

Madaras, Lynda, and Area Madaras. *My Body, My Self for Girls*. Rev. 2nd ed. New York, NY: Newmarket Press, 2007.

Middleman, Amy B., and Kate Gruenwald Pfeifer. *American Medical Association Boy's Guide to Becoming a Teen*. San Francisco, CA: Jossey-Bass, 2006.

Middleman, Amy B., and Kate Gruenwald Pfeifer. *American Medical Association Girl's Guide to Becoming a Teen*. San Francisco, CA: Jossey-Bass, 2006.

Spilsbury, Louise. *Me, Myself, and I: All About Sex and Puberty*. Hauppauge, NY: Barron's, 2010.

Thomas, Isabel. *Why Do I Have Periods? Menstruation and Puberty (Inside My Body)*. Chicago, IL: Raintree, 2011.

BIBLIOGRAPHY

American Academy of Pediatrics. "Obesity's Impact on Teen Health." HealthyChildren.org, May 26, 2011. Retrieved November 3, 2011 (http://www.healthychildren.org/English/health-issues/conditions/obesity/pages/Obesitys-Impact-on-Teen-Health.aspx).

Bolyn, Michelle. "What Are the Symptoms of Too Much Stress on Teens?" Livestrong.com, April 28, 2010. Retrieved November 4, 2011 (http://livestrong.com/article/113091-symptoms-much-stress-teens).

Center for Young Women's Health, Children's Hospital Boston. "Endometriosis: A Guide for Teens." April 8, 2010. Retrieved November 3, 2011 (http://www.youngwomenshealth.org/endoinfo.html).

Centers for Disease Control and Prevention. "Fact Sheets—Underage Drinking—Alcohol." July 20, 2010. Retrieved November 3, 2011 (http://www.cdc.gov/alcohol/fact-sheets/underage-drinking.htm).

Centers for Disease Control and Prevention. "Health Effects of Cigarette Smoking—Smoking & Tobacco Use." March 21, 2011. Retrieved November 3, 2011 (http://www.cdc.gov/tobacco/data_statistics/fact_sheets/health_effects/effects_cig_smoking/index.htm).

Cole, Gary W., and Craig A. Manifold. "Jock Itch." eMedicineHealth.com, 2011. Retrieved November 3, 2011 (http://www.emedicinehealth.com/jock_itch/article_em.htm).

Loulan, JoAnn, and Bonnie Worthen. *Period: A Girl's Guide*. Minnetonka, MN: Book Peddlers, 2001.

Macnair, Trisha. "Body Odour." BBC Health. Retrieved November 3, 2011 (http://www.bbc.co.uk/health/physical_health/conditions/bodyodour2.shtml).

National Institute of Mental Health. "Eating Disorders." NIH publication No. 11-4901, revised 2011. Retrieved November 3, 2011

(http://www.nimh.nih.gov/health/publications/eating-disorders/
eating-disorders.pdf).

National Sleep Foundation. "Teens and Sleep." Retrieved November
3, 2011 (http://www.sleepfoundation.org/article/sleep-topics/
teens-and-sleep).

Nemours Foundation. "Testicular Injuries." KidsHealth.org,
September 2010. Retrieved November 3, 2011 (http://kidshealth
.org/teen/safety/first_aid/testicular_injuries.html).

Nemours Foundation. "Why Do I Get Acne?" KidsHealth.org,
January 2011. Retrieved November 3, 2011 (http://kidshealth
.org/teen/your_body/skin_stuff/acne.html).

Nemours Foundation. "Why Is My Voice Changing?" KidsHealth.org,
May 2010. Retrieved November 3, 2011 (http://kidshealth.org/
teen/sexual_health/guys/voice_changing.html).

Office on Women's Health. "Anorexia Nervosa Fact Sheet."
WomensHealth.gov, June 15, 2009. Retrieved November 2, 2011
(http://www.womenshealth.gov/publications/our%2Dpublications/
fact-sheet/anorexia-nervosa.cfm).

Office on Women's Health. "Getting Your Period—Your Changing
Body." GirlsHealth.gov, October 13, 2010. Retrieved November
3, 2011 (http://www.girlshealth.gov/body/period/index.cfm).

PBS.org. "Interviews—Mary Carskadon—Inside the Teenage Brain."
Frontline, January 31, 2002. Retrieved November 3, 2011 (http://
www.pbs.org/wgbh/pages/frontline/shows/teenbrain/interviews/
carskadon.html).

WebMD.com. "Yeast Infections: Symptoms, Treatments, Causes."
June 8, 2010. Retrieved November 3, 2011 (http://www.webmd
.com/tc/vaginal-yeast-infections-topic-overview)

INDEX

About the Author

Serena Gander-Howser is an educator who works with at-risk middle school students in Brooklyn, New York. Her class topics have included current events, self-expression, conflict resolution, and character education. She has worked in the education field for more than ten years.

Photo Credits

Cover © istockphoto.com/Neustockimages; p. 5 © istockphoto.com/ Monkey Business Images; p. 7 © istockphoto.com/Sashkin; p. 8 Dorling Kindersley/the Agency Collection/Getty Images; p. 10 Andy Reynolds/Taxi/Getty Images; pp. 12, 20 Peter Gardner/SPL/Custom Medical Stock Photo; p. 13 Brand X Pictures/Thinkstock; p. 15 Martyn F. Chillmaid/Photo Researchers, Inc.; p. 21 istockphoto/Thinkstock; p. 23 Shutterstock.com/szefei; p. 27 Hans Neleman/Taxi/Getty Images; p. 28 Comstock/Jupiterimages/Getty Images/Thinkstock; p. 30 Catherine Lender/Stone+/Getty Images; p. 34 © istockphoto .com/Ana Abejon; p. 37 © agefotostock/SuperStock; p. 39 Camille Tokerud/Iconica/Getty Images; p. 41 Shutterstock.com/Aleksandr Markin; p. 45 Shutterstock.com/CandyBox Images; p. 48 istockphoto/Thinkstock; cover (inset), p. 1 (inset) (lung illustration) © istockphoto.com/bubaone; cover (background graphic), interior graphic (frame) © istockphoto.com/liquidplanet; interior graphic (ECG waves) © istockphoto.com/linearcurves.

Designer: Brian Garvey; Editor: Andrea Sclarow Paskoff;
Photo Researcher: Marty Levick